DISEASES *of* THE EAR

A Pocket Atlas

This Pocket Atlas was produced
with the assistance of a generous educational grant from
Starkey Laboratories, Inc.

DISEASES *of* THE EAR
A Pocket Atlas

MICHAEL HAWKE, M.D.

Professor of Otolaryngology and Pathology, University of Toronto
Chief of Otolaryngology,
St. Joseph's Hospital, Toronto, Ontario, Canada

ANDREW McCOMBE, M.B.

TWJ Fellow, Department of Otolaryngology,
University of Toronto

1995 MANTICORE COMMUNICATIONS INC.

NOTICE

The authors and publisher have done all they can to ensure that the care which may be recommended in this book reflects the best current practices and standards (this includes choice of medication and dosage). As research, regulations, and clinical practices are constantly changing you are encouraged to check all product information sheets from all medication packages. If in doubt about anything in this book or on the product information sheets, contact your personal physician for advice on the proper procedure.

Printed in Canada

ISBN 1-896251-02-1

Contents

To Bill Austin,
whose strong support for continuing medical education
made this atlas possible.

Introduction

The human ear is the organ responsible for hearing. It is composed of three parts: the outer, the middle and the inner ears. The outer ear consists of all that lies lateral to the tympanic membrane and includes the pinna and the external auditory meatus. This part of the ear serves to "capture and funnel" sound waves down to the tympanic membrane. The convolutions of the pinna also act to provide resonances to the incident sound which are direction dependent. This function provides important information for sound localization. The middle ear is an air-filled space lying between the tympanic membrane and the bony wall of the inner ear. It contains the three ossicles: the malleus, the incus and the stapes and two muscles: the stapedius muscle and the tensor tympani muscle. The middle ear acts as an impedance matcher or "transformer", converting the low pressure, high amplitude airborne vibrations into low amplitude, higher pressure fluid vibrations in the cochlea. The two muscles are stimulated by loud sounds and have a role in protecting the cochlea from the damaging effects of noise. The inner ear is fluid-filled and is made up of the cochlea, the utricle, the saccule and the three semicircular canals. The cochlea is the part of the inner ear that is concerned with hearing; the other parts providing important information for balance. The cochlea contains specialized hair cells which are sensitive to the vibrations in the fluid of the inner ear. They convert this mechanical energy, and the information it contains, into neuro-electrical signals which are passed via the acoustic nerve to the brain where it is perceived as sound.

The human ear is sensitive to a broad range of sound frequencies (20 - 20000 Hz) but it is most sensitive to those sounds that occur around the same frequencies as human speech. This is not surprising, as speech and communication are of fundamental importance to the continued development of mankind.

Adequate hearing is essential in the development of speech in an infant. It is necessary for education and academic development and it is paramount for normal social and domestic interactions at all stages of life.

For these reasons it is essential that the hearing of any individual be optimized. Hearing loss may be described as conductive or sensorineural. In the latter there is damage to the neuro-sensory elements. Sensorineural hearing loss is invariably unresponsive to any form of medical or surgical treatment although the individual may gain substantial assistance from appropriate amplification (hearing aid). In the former there is failure of the normal transmission of sound from the environment to the cochlea. Although this type of hearing loss may also benefit from amplification, it is often amenable to medical or surgical therapy. Nearly every condition that affects the external or middle ears will have some effect on hearing. In many conditions hearing loss will not be the main symptom and in some cases there will be no effect on hearing at all. However, there are often other symptoms such as earache and discharge which can be most unpleasant.

Prompt recognition and accurate diagnosis are the first requirements for appropriate treatment. This book aims to help in this role by providing an illustrated reference to some of the more commonly encountered otological conditions and a brief guide to their management.

Embryology

The three portions of the ear develop separately. There is little to see before the third week but development is almost complete by the end of the first trimester (14 weeks). First to appear is a cellular ectodermal thickening at the cranial end of the developing embryo at the end of the third week. This is the otic placode and over the next two weeks it slowly invaginates to become the membranous labyrinth. The surrounding mesenchyme ossifies to form the bony labyrinth during weeks nine to twenty-three.

The eustachian tube and the middle ear develop from the tubotympanic recess, an extension of the first pharyngeal pouch, which extends laterally between the developing internal and external ears. Commencing in the fourth week, the cartilage of the first and second arches gives rise to the ossicles. Finally the external ear and the external auditory canal develop from six cartilaginous hillocks situated around the dorsal/lateral aspect of the first branchial groove: three from the first arch and three from the second. This commences between the fourth and sixth weeks of gestation.

Although formation of the "ear" is largely complete by about the 14th week, and it is probably functional soon after, the "middle ear cleft" and the external auditory meatus are filled with mesenchymal and ectodermal material respectively until the last few weeks of gestation when they finally canalize to produce the "normal" anatomy.

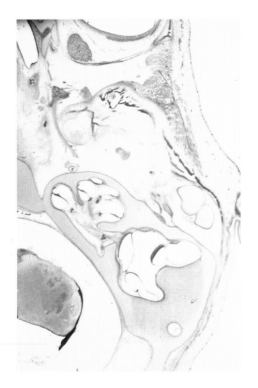

Figure 1.1 Cross-section of the skull of a
12 week fetus
This section of a twelve-week-old fetal skull demon-
strates the early formation of the inner, middle and
external ears.

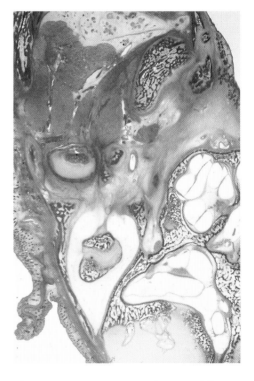

Figure 1.2 Cross-section of a 20 week fetus
The appearance at this stage is very close to the adult
form. All three parts of the ear are recognizable, as are
the ossicles in the middle ear and the organ of Corti
in the cochlea.

Tools

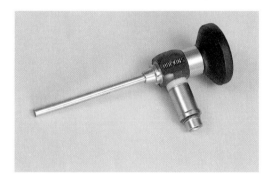

Figure 2.1 Hopkins Rod Tele-Otoscope
With the advent of the "Hopkins rod lens system" (named after its English inventor Professor Harold Hopkins of Reading, England) in the 1960s, medical instruments have been developed to take advantage of this revolutionary optical technology. The Hopkins Rod Tele-Otoscope is the ideal tool for visualizing and photographing the external canal and tympanic membrane and in fact allows a wider field of view than the standard otoscopes. All of the photographs of the external auditory canal, tympanic membrane, and middle ear in this book were taken with the Karl Storz Hopkins Rod Tele-Otoscope shown here.

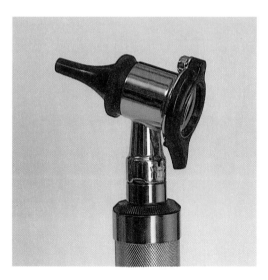

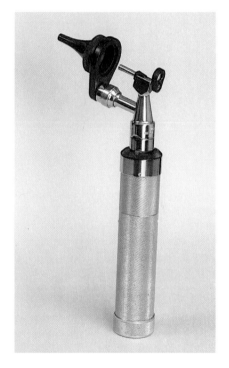

Figure 2.2 Operating (Open head) Otoscope
The body of the operating otoscope is open and the rear lens is smaller and mobile. This configuration allows the clinician to use one hand to manipulate instruments into the ear canal and perform minor procedures, such as cleaning wax, myringotomy or biopsy.

Figure 2.3 Welch Allyn Diagnostic Otoscope
This instrument is the work horse for otological examination. The handpiece contains a rechargeable battery power supply. The head contains a small bulb for illumination and the speculum allows access to the external ear canal. The rear lens provides low power magnification of the visualized structures. The closed head allows the pressure within the external auditory canal to be varied by squeezing the attached soft rubber bulb. This allows assessment of tympanic membrane mobility (pneumatic otoscopy).

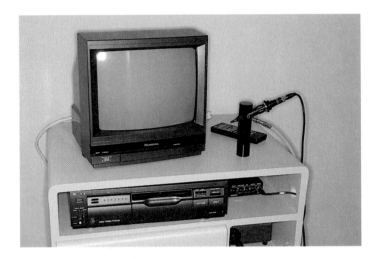

Figure 2.4 Starkey Video-Otoscope

These slides show a modern video-viewing system. The system utilizes a short Hopkins rod, a small video camera, a TV monitor and finally a video capture printing device that allows still photographs to be taken of any interesting findings. There is no doubt that this is a useful tool for both clinician and patient education and provides an unparalleled opportunity for further visual exposure to the huge range of aural pathologies, most of which rely on visualization for their diagnosis.

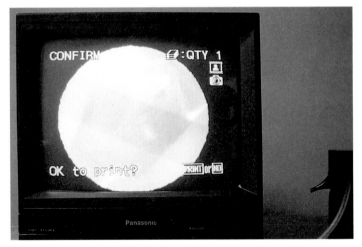

The Pinna

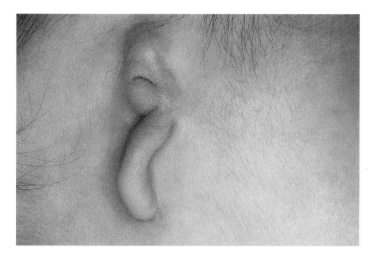

Figure 3.1 Microtia

This term implies a failure in the development of the external ear and usually the external auditory canal. Severity is variable and does not necessarily indicate any problem of the middle or inner ears. There is, however, a frequent association with other congenital abnormalities. Reconstruction is rarely satisfactory but bone-anchored hearing aids and prosthesis have given excellent results.

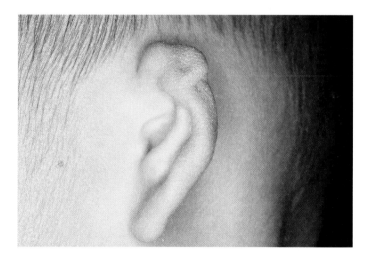

Figure 3.2 Atresia of the external ear

There is a mild developmental abnormality of the pinna and there has been a complete failure of canalization of the external auditory meatus. Surgical reconstruction may be successful in the presence of a relatively normal middle ear.

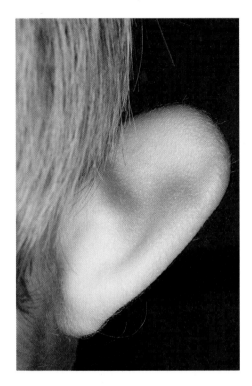

Figure 3.3 Prominent ears
This is probably the most common deformity of the
pinna and is due to a failure of development of
the normal anti-helical fold. Outstanding ears are
inherited by means of an autosomal dominant gene
with variable expression. This deformity may result
in teasing at school and occasionally disturbs the
parents more than the child. There are no adverse
effects on hearing.

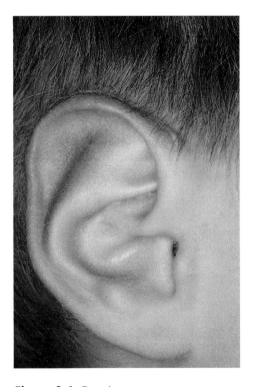

Figure 3.4 Prominent ears
A pinnaplasty or otoplasty is a cosmetic operation
that involves surgical manipulation of the cartilage to
recreate the anti-helical fold. It is usually performed
just before school age.

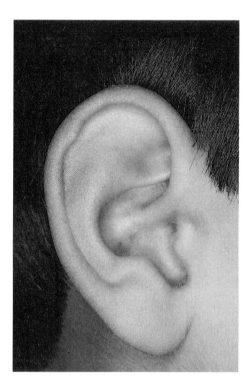

Figure 3.5 Darwin's tubercle
This small cartilaginous protuberance is also common and is usually situated along the concave edge of the postero-superior helix but may occasionally project posteriorly. It has no particular significance.

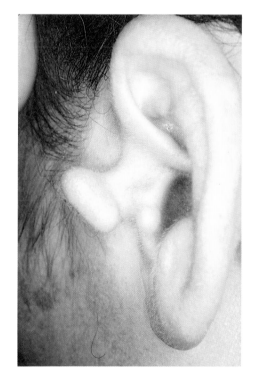

Figure 3.6 Preauricular tag
These small accessory skin tags are most often found just anterior to the upper border of the tragus and represent a failure of the normal development of one of the original embryological hillocks.

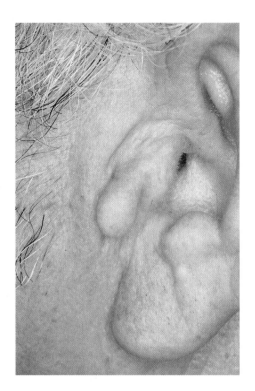

Figure 3.7 Accessory auricle

Occasionally, skin tags may be larger and possess a cartilage core; receiving the title of "accessory auricle". If unsightly they may warrant surgical removal.

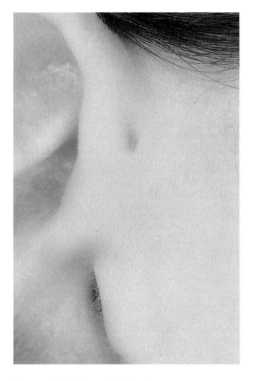

Figure 3.8 Preauricular sinus

These may occur as shallow pits or deep sinuses, again as a result of failure in the fusion of parts of the embryological hillocks. They are most frequently located just in front of the anterior crus of the helix.

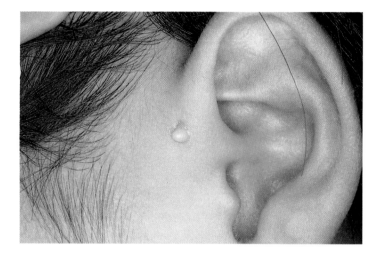

Figure 3.9 Preauricular sinus

Although rarely troublesome if shallow, if they are deep they may be prone to repetitive infections. If this is the case surgical removal should be offered. The whole tract, which will often extend all the way down to the tragus, must be removed in its entirety.

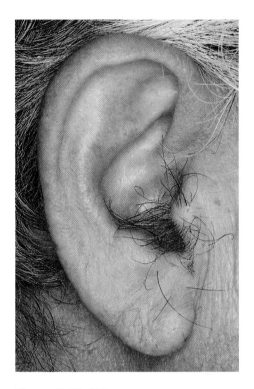

Figure 3.10 Hairy tragus

This condition is more often found in men than women. Its practical significance lies in the fact that similar thick hairs are usually also found lining the lateral part of the external auditory meatus. This can interfere with the normal external migration of wax and debris leading to their accumulation in the ear canal.

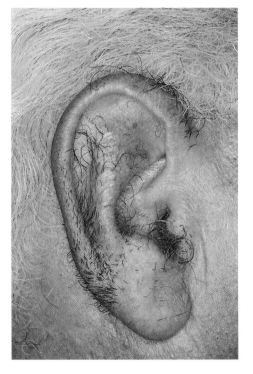

Figure 3.11 Hairy ear

In some cases hair growth is so florid that the whole ear is covered. This, however, occurs only in males as it is inherited as a Y-linked trait.

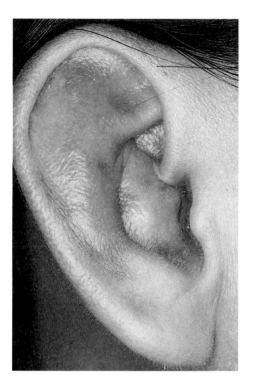

Figure 3.12 Haematoma

This is usually the result of blunt trauma to the ear. The blood collects in the subperiosteal plane and, if not treated, will lead to an unsightly thickening of the ear: "cauliflower ear". A haematoma is rarely found on the medial surface as the skin in this area is more mobile on the subcutaneous tissue.

Figure 3.13 Haematoma – button

Treatment is by the aspiration of the haematoma and the application of a pressure dressing. In this case a button has been sutured through the pinna to maintain pressure in the concha.

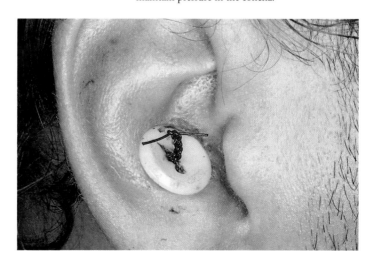

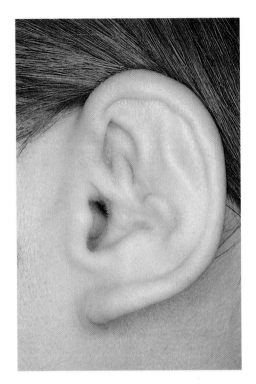

Figure 3.14 Cauliflower ear
Failure to treat this problem adequately leads to the all too familiar deformity of cauliflower ear.

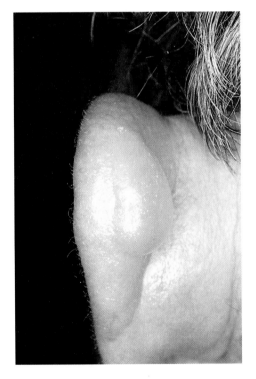

Figure 3.15 Frostbite
Exposure to extremely low temperatures may damage the skin of the pinna. The result, which is termed a frostbite, is similar in its effects to a second degree burn.

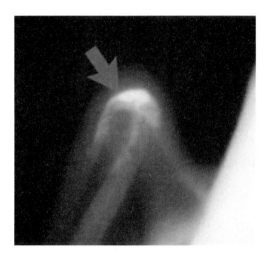

Figure 3.16 Calcified auricular cartilage (bony pinna)
Frostbite may cause damage to the underlying auricular cartilage which results in the gradual deposition of calcium within it, producing a rigid "bony" hard pinna.

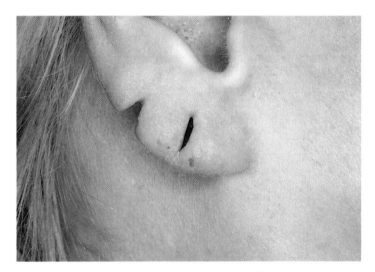

Figure 3.17 Split lobule and elongated earring hole
This irregular deformity is not uncommon amongst the wearers of earrings. It results when an earring is pulled, usually by a child or an assailant. It is a relatively simple procedure to repair but may preclude the future wearing of earrings. Note the elongation of the earring hole which is the result of wearing excessively heavy earrings.

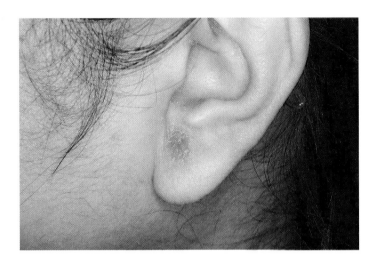

Figure 3.18 Contact dermatitis
This usually occurs as the result of contact sensitivity to the nickel contained in cheap jewelry. The tract may also become secondarily infected. Treatment is simple by avoidance, the application of a topical steroid cream, and the wearing of more expensive jewelry!

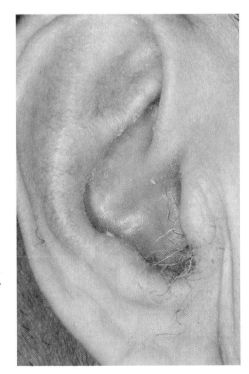

Figure 3.19 Ear mold contact dermatitis
In some unfortunate individuals a contact sensitivity may develop to materials used in the manufacture of the ear mold. These patients frequently complain of persistent itching and display an irritated, shiny, erythematous appearance to the concha, as seen in this patient. Treatment involves topical steroids and the fitting of a hypo-allergenic mold.

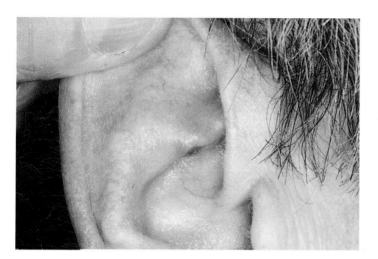

Figure 3.20 Ear mold ulceration
Pressure from an ill-fitting ear mold may lead to a painful superficial ulceration
of the skin of the pinna, in this case of the anti-tragus.

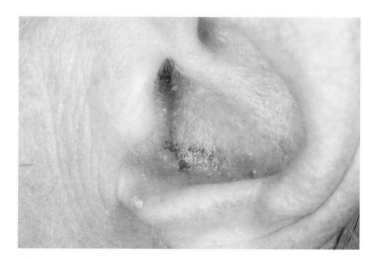

Figure 3.21 Neurodermatitis
The skin of the concha may become itchy for no clinically apparent reason during times of "stress". This leads to vigorous scratching and marked excoriation
of the "itchy" area. This phenomenon is termed "neurodermatitis" and may ulti-
mately lead to a chronic bacterial or fungal local dermatitis.

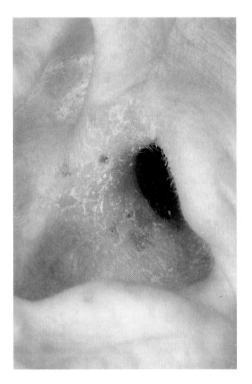

Figure 3.22 Localized infective dermatitis (conchitis)

This slide shows a localized staphylococcal dermatitis caused by a combination of poor local hygiene and pressure from a hearing aid ear mold.

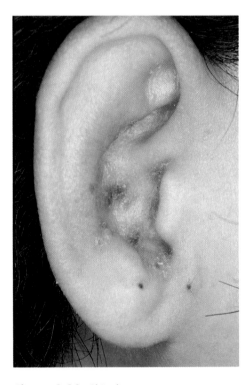

Figure 3.23 Shingles

The Herpes Zoster virus survives in the ganglia of sensory nerves and may become active for many reasons. When it does so, it causes an acute and painful skin vesicular infection localized to the area of skin subserved by the affected sensory nerve. In this case it is affecting the small sensory portion of the facial nerve. If the motor part of the nerve is affected at the same time, and a facial palsy results, the condition is eponymously called the "Ramsay Hunt syndrome".

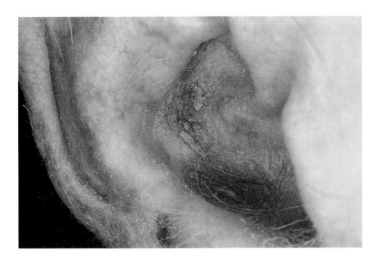

Figure 3.24 Neglect keratosis

Normal skin is a multi-layered structure that is constantly replaced from an active basal layer while the outer layer of keratinized squames is constantly shed, usually as a result of friction from clothes or personal toilet. If this does not occur with the passage of time and contact with the air, the accumulated keratin will discolour and become dark. Although, at first sight, this resembles a seborrhoeic keratosis, it can be removed easily with a little rubbing to reveal healthy pink skin beneath.

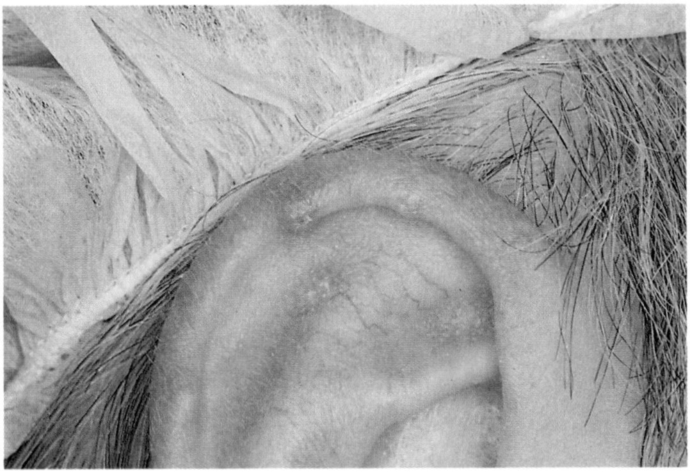

Figure 3.25 Chondrodermatitis helicis nodularis

This exquisitely tender nodule is the result of degeneration of the underlying helical cartilage. This leads to ulceration and breakdown of the overlying skin as the body makes efforts to extrude the damaged cartilage. Local excision is curative.

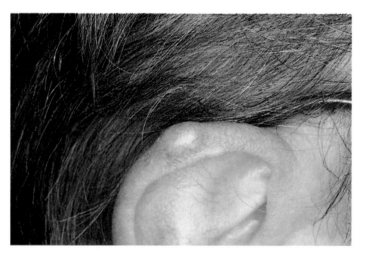

Figure 3.26 Gouty tophus

Gout is a metabolic disorder of urate metabolism and can lead to the deposition of urate crystals in various parts of the body. Although gouty tophi of the external ear are uncommon, they should be included in the differential diagnosis of painful nodules on the external ear. Typically they feel gritty and occur on the helix.

External Ear Canal

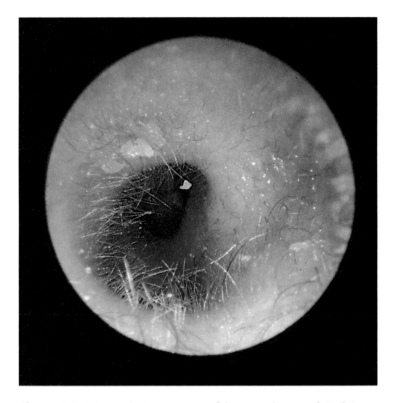

Figure 4.1 The cartilaginous portion of the external ear canal (Right)
The external ear canal is divided into two parts: a medial or bony portion (two thirds) and a lateral or cartilaginous portion (one third). The cartilaginous portion of the canal is lined by a thick hair-bearing skin which is rich in sebaceous and ceruminous glands. It is supported by a surrounding cartilaginous skeleton.

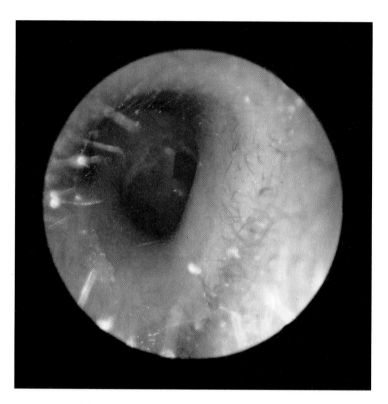

Figure 4.2 The bony portion of the external ear canal (Left)
The medial or bony portion of the external auditory canal is surrounded by bone.
The skin lining it is thin and contains no adnexal structures. The medial
limit of the external auditory canal is defined by the tympanic membrane which
lies obliquely.

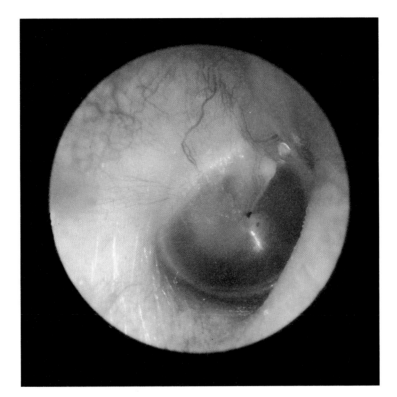

Figure 4.3 Epithelial migration 1

Unlike the rest of the body, in the deep external auditory meatus the superficial keratin squames cannot be shed by friction. To circumvent this potential problem, the external canal has a self-cleansing mechanism. The superficial layer of the epithelium lining the deep external canal is slowly carried laterally by the mysterious and elegant process of epithelial migration. In this slide an ink dot has been applied to the center of the tympanic membrane.

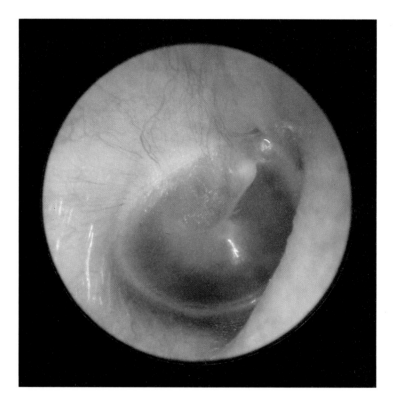

Figure 4.4 Epithelial migration 2
The epithelium on the surface of the tympanic membrane moves in a radial
direction until it reaches the walls of the canal. This is seen in this slide made two
months later.

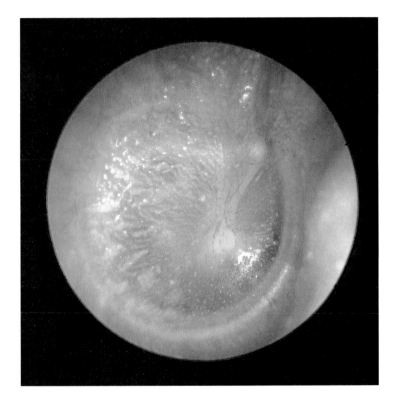

Figure 4.5 Epithelial migration – keratin patches
This radial movement can sometimes be seen without the aid of an ink dot by
the presence of radially orientated patches of thickened keratin as seen here on an
otherwise normal eardrum.

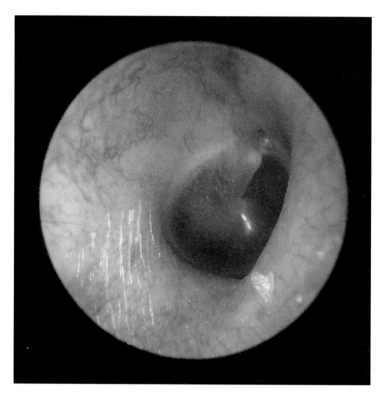

Figure 4.6 Epithelial migration 4
Upon reaching the canal wall the skin migrates laterally as seen in this slide taken after a further two months.

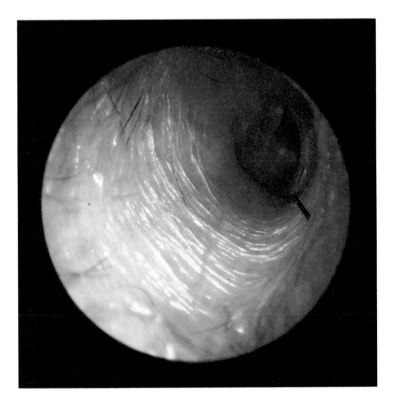

Figure 4.7 Wrinkles of the external canal 5
As the skin migrates laterally it eventually reaches resistance in the form of the
hairs of the cartilaginous portion of the canal. This "traffic jam" leads to a piling up
of the epithelium and the development of the wrinkles as seen.

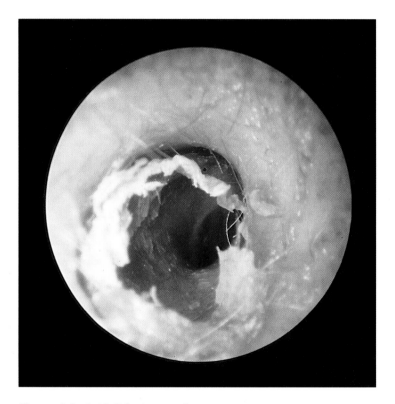

Figure 4.8 Epithelial migration 6

Finally, the migrating sheet of keratin squames mix with the ceruminous secretions and the whole complex becomes "earwax". Movements, particularly talking and chewing, are transmitted through the cartilaginous canal and help to loosen the wax which finally leaves the canal spontaneously or with the aid of a judicious small finger or cotton-tipped applicator!

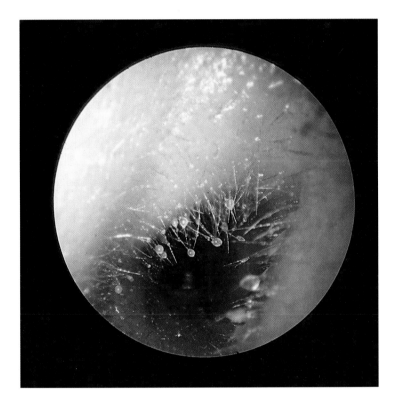

Figure 4.9 Earwax
"Wax" is a mixture of desquamated keratin, debris and the secretions of the
ceruminous glands. The ceruminous glands are located in the lateral hair-bearing
portion of the canal and secrete their product around the base of the hairs.

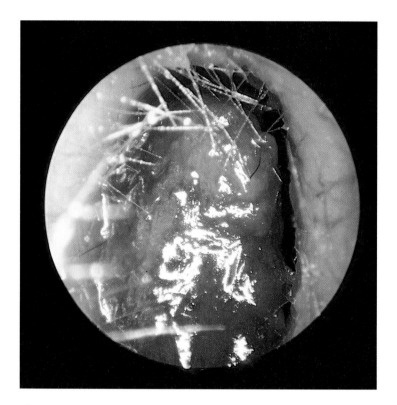

Figure 4.10 Earwax
The actual appearance of the wax in any individual depends on the type of cerumen secreted, the amount of keratin and the presence of any debris. However, cerumen is secreted in two basic forms. The moist, soft, brown form (Wet form) shown here is the most common.

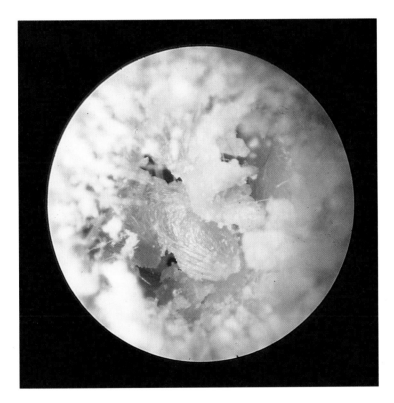

Figure 4.11 Earwax
The alternative form of cerumen is the dry or "Oriental" form. This tends to be of light color and is obviously dry and flaky. As its name implies, it is more common in people of oriental origin.

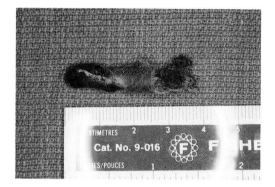

Figure 4.12 Earwax

Approximately 10 percent of adults may develop such an accumulation of wax that the canal is occluded and a mild conductive hearing loss results. This appears to be more common in people who habitually use cotton-tipped applicators. Removal may be performed by suction under direct vision or by syringing, in which case softening with a cerumenolytic may first be required.

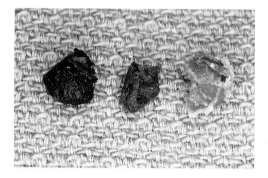

Figure 4.13 Earwax

There is great variation in the color of normal earwax from golden yellow to almost black as shown here.

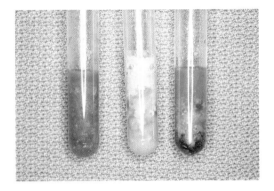

Figure 4.14 Ceruminolytics 1
The most effective ceruminolytics appear to have an
aqueous base as shown by this slide in which there
is obvious swelling and dissolution of the wax.
(From the left: sodium bicarbonate, hydrogen perox-
ide, distilled water.)

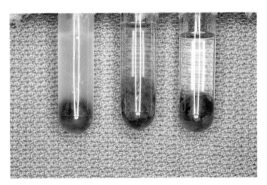

Figure 4.15 Ceruminolytics 2
In marked contrast those with an oil base appear much
less effective. (From the left: Cerumol, Cerumenex, olive
oil.)

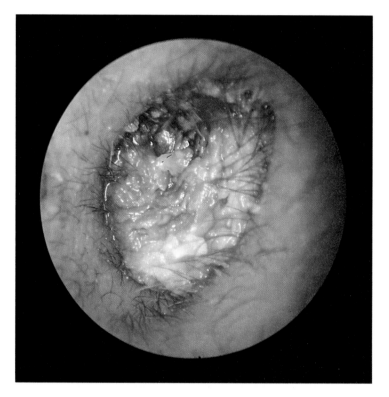

Figure 4.16 Keratosis obturans 1

In this condition there is a failure of the normal process of epithelial migration.
The result is an accumulation of desquamated keratinous squames in the deep part
of the external auditory meatus.

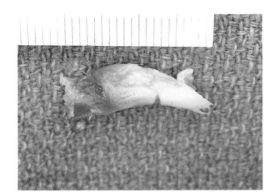

Figure 4.17 Keratosis obturans 2

This shows the typical appearance of a keratin plug after its removal. The typical white cheesy appearance of fresh keratin is seen in the deep portion of the plug. Although the lateral part of the plug has all the appearances of normal wax, it is in fact keratin that has undergone a chemical reaction after prolonged exposure to the air (oxidation) and turned brown.

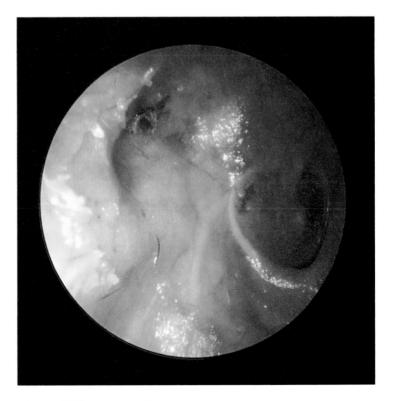

Figure 4.18 Keratosis obturans 3

The presence of the keratin plug sets up a low grade inflammatory response in the canal. Various inflammatory mediators are released and a process of adjacent bone erosion results. This can lead to a widening of the bony canal or even, as in this case after five years, an "auto-mastoidectomy". The diagnosis is confirmed by the presence of an intact, and usually normal, tympanic membrane.

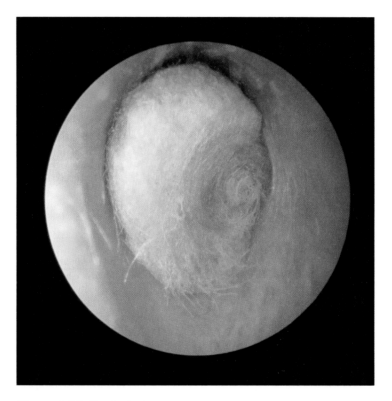

Figure 4.19 Foreign body 1

A plethora of objects may find their way into the external auditory meatus, more often in children than adults. Symptoms will vary depending on the size and nature of the foreign body. In this case, a very common finding, a plug of cotton wool was seen completely asymptomatically in the deep meatus.

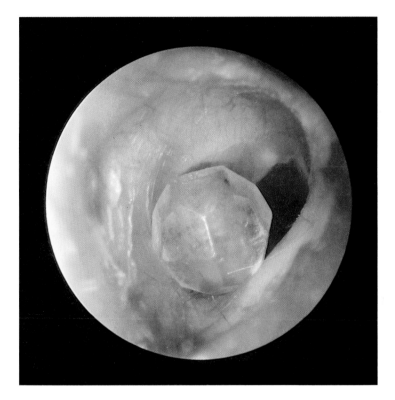

Figure 4.20 Foreign body 2
A plastic bead was found in this young child. A general anaesthetic was required
for removal due to the lack of patient cooperation. This is rarely, if ever, required for
foreign bodies in adults. Syringing is also often useful for foreign body removal.

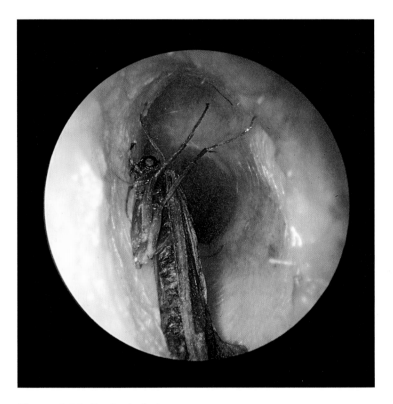

Figure 4.21   Foreign body 3

Other symptoms include a conductive hearing loss if the foreign body occludes the meatus, pain and bleeding if there has been local trauma, and, in this case, an acute otitis externa produced by local irritation of the meatal skin. The underlying cause for the problem only became apparent after treatment of the secondary otitis externa.

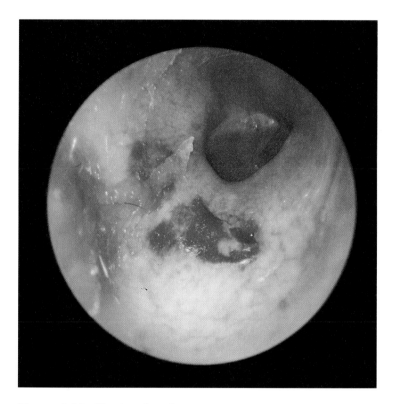

Figure 4.22 Abrasion of canal
The epithelium lining the external auditory meatus is thin and easily damaged.
An abrasion is easily produced either by medical cleaning of the canal or, more
frequently, as in this case by the use of a cotton-tipped applicator.

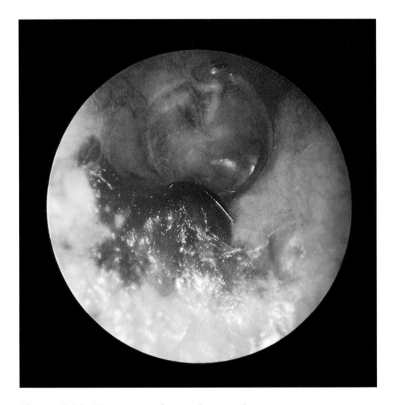

Figure 4.23 Haematoma of external ear canal
With really aggressive use of the cotton-tipped applicator, evidence of more severe
trauma can be found. In this case a large canal haematoma has been the result. This
can precipitate an otitis externa.

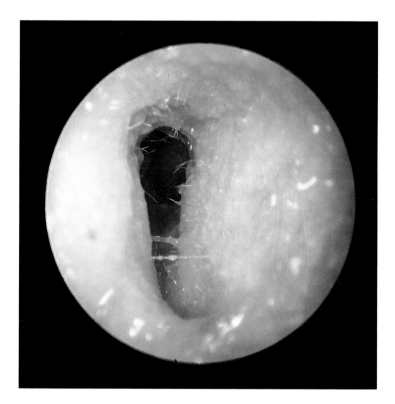

Figure 4.24 Otitis externa 1
Acute otitis externa is an inflammatory condition affecting the epithelium lining
the external auditory meatus. It most often occurs as an acute infective dermatitis
with Pseudomonas aeruginosa as one of the most common infecting organisms.
The early stages shown here are most often characterized by severe otalgia. There is
visible swelling of the epithelium giving this typical follicular appearance and early
serous discharge.

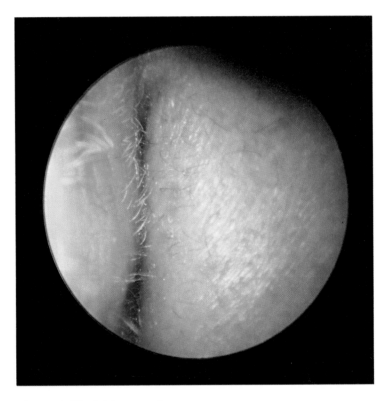

Figure 4.25 Otitis externa 2

As the condition progresses there is often progressive swelling of the epithelium
lining such that the lumen may be occluded.

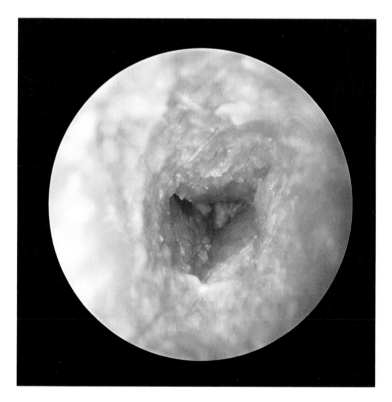

Figure 4.26 Otitis externa 3

The inflammatory process inevitably leads to a hyperkeratosis and a failure of the normal process of migration so that there is also a buildup of keratinous debris in the canal. This acts as a further inflammatory stimulant and perpetuates the condition. For this reason thorough aural toilet is an essential part of the treatment of this condition.

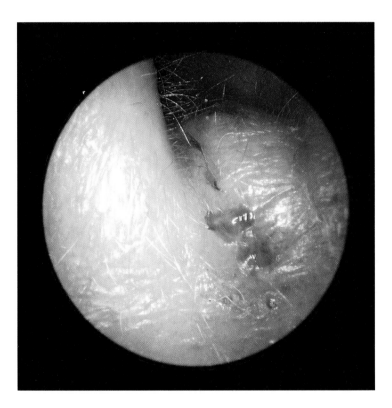

Figure 4.27 Otitis externa 4 - Furuncle
A furuncle or pimple is included in the description of otitis externa as an acute localized form. It is an acute staphylococcal abscess and occurs only in the hair-bearing part of the canal. It is acutely painful but is usually self-resolving in a few days.

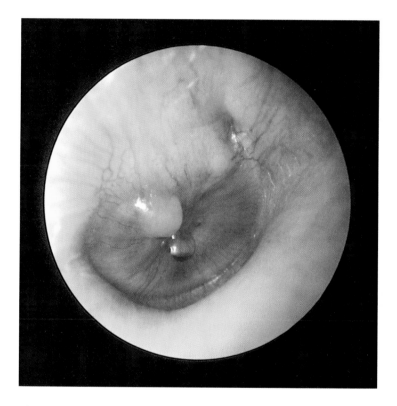

Figure 4.28 Bullous myringitis

This is another localized form of external otitis. Caused by a virus, it leads to bullous eruptions on the tympanic membrane and skin of the deep canal. Excruciating pain is the prominent feature but the condition is self-resolving after a few days and only symptomatic treatment is required.

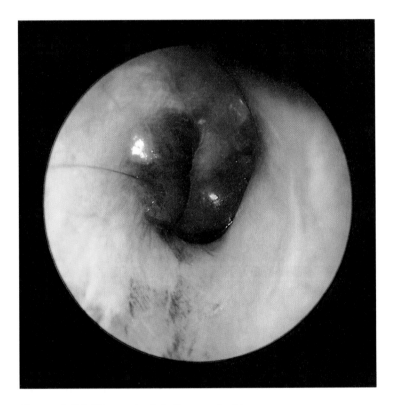

Figure 4.29 Haemorrhagic bullous myringitis
If the condition is particularly severe, haemorrhage is frequently seen in close association with the bulla.

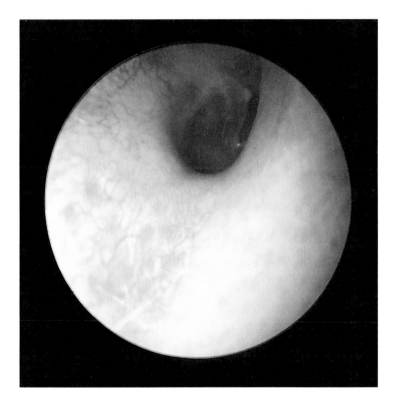

Figure 4.30 Chronic otitis externa

This is a common condition. Patients frequently complain of itchiness and irritation and less often of pain and discharge. Earwax is rarely seen while the condition is active.

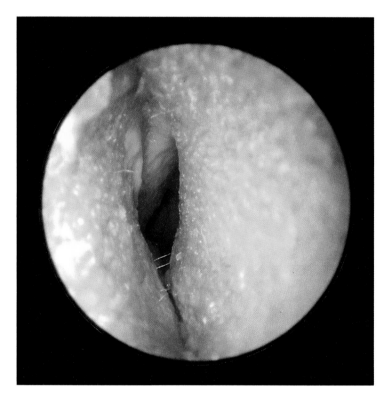

Figure 4.31 Chronic hypertrophic otitis externa

Frequently the persistence of the condition leads to a fibrosis and irreversible thickening of the epithelium lining the external canal. This may be sufficient to compromise the lumen of the canal.

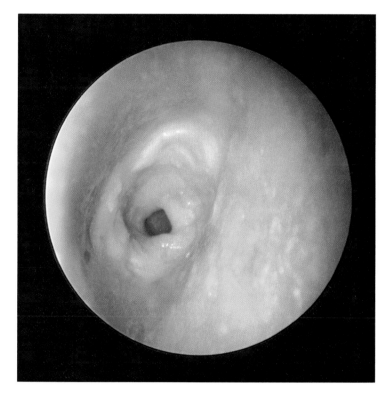

Figure 4.32 Chronic otitis externa 2

This condition also shows a frequent buildup of keratin debris with its inflammatory properties. Treatment again involves meticulous toilet and the use of topical
antibiotic/steroid combinations.

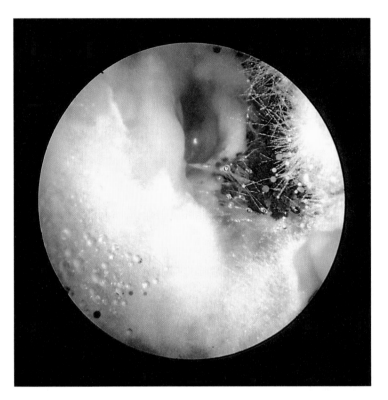

Figure 4.33 Otomycosis 1

Otitis externa, particularly when chronic and treated by frequent antibiotic drops, can become complicated by a fungal superinfection. This case shows the classic features of aspergillus niger with fluffy fungal hyphae and black spores. Treatment again demands meticulous toilet and topical antifungal agents.

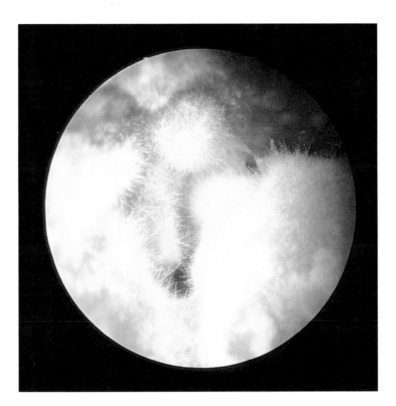

Figure 4.34 Otomycosis 2

In this patient the hyphae are particularly prominent and there are no visible spores. This probably represents an early stage in the germination of the fungus.

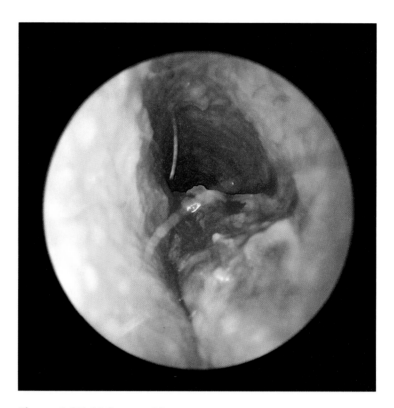

Figure 4.35 Malignant otitis externa

This life-threatening condition is essentially an osteitis of the temporal bone caused, almost invariably, by Pseudomonas. Typical patients are elderly diabetics who present with severe otalgia and display exuberant granulation tissue in the bony canal as shown here. The high mortality is usually due to lower cranial nerve palsies and consequent aspiration pneumonia.

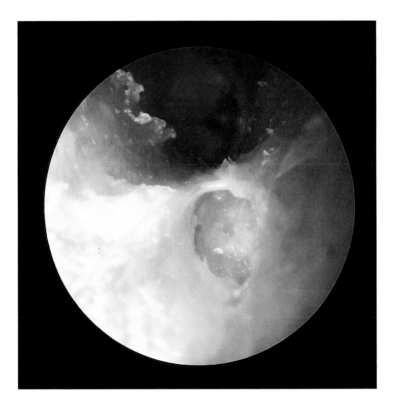

Figure 4.36 Osteitis of the tympanic bone
Osteitis, the presence of exposed bone and surrounding inflammation, as shown here, is an essential requirement for the diagnosis of malignant otitis externa. This condition may also occur following radiotherapy to the head and neck, in severe, non-malignant, otitis externa and in keratosis obturans.

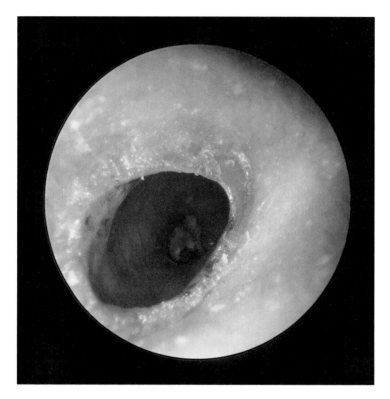

Figure 4.37 Stenosis of the external auditory meatus 1
Repeated infections or trauma to the external auditory meatus can lead to circum-ferential ulceration and subsequent granulation tissue formation. If healing should occur, scar contracture can lead to a web-like stenosis of the canal.

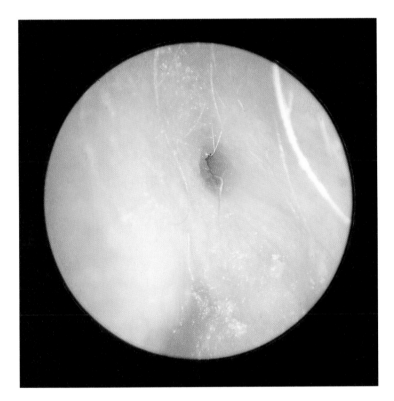

Figure 4.38 Stenosis of the external auditory meatus 2
The condition may become so severe that there is almost complete occlusion of the canal. This can lead to problems with both hearing and epithelial migration.

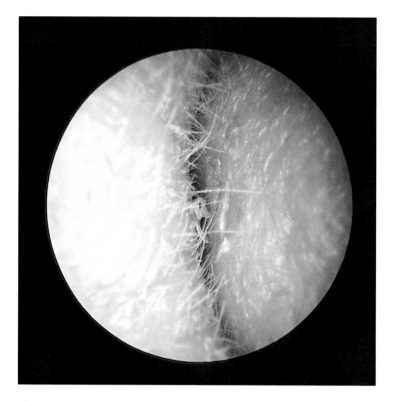

Figure 4.39 Collapsing canal

The ear canal may be compromised for other reasons. This finding is not infrequent, particularly in the elderly population, and results from a deficiency of the supporting cartilage. The collapse may be aggravated by pressure from a pair of headphones thus leading to an erroneous estimation of the hearing threshold.

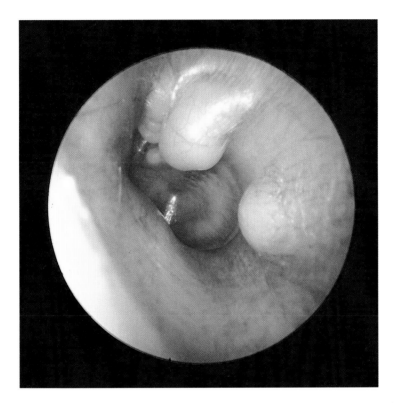

Figure 4.40 Bony exostoses

Another cause of compromise of the external canal are bony exostoses. These rarely cause problems with either hearing or migration. They are due to excessive bony growth as a result of stimulation of the canal periostium by frequent exposure to cold, usually from swimming.

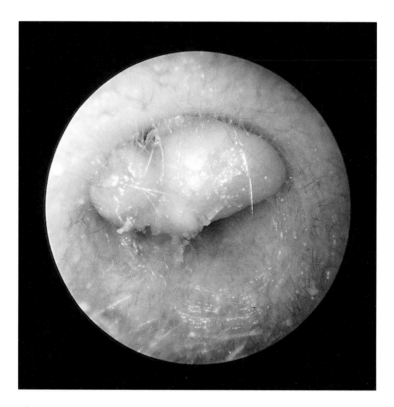

Figure 4.41 Osteoma

In contrast to exostoses which are common, osteoma are rare benign tumors of the temporal bone, usually lying in the external ear canal. If they occur they are more likely to warrant surgical removal as they more frequently compromise the canal.

Middle Ear

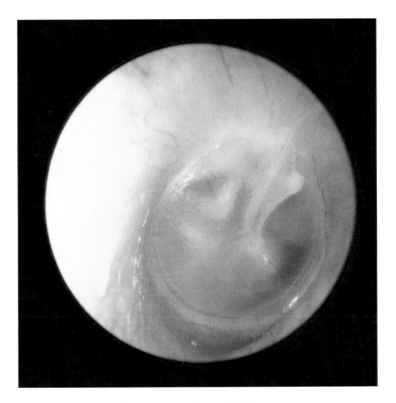

Figure 5.1 Normal tympanic membrane (Right)

The tympanic membrane is a greyish translucent ovoid membrane that lies obliquely to the long axis of the external canal. It provides a semi-transparent window to the middle ear. The handle of the malleus can be clearly seen centrally. The long process of the incus and the incudo-stapedial joint are well demonstrated behind the postero-superior quadrant of this tympanic membrane.

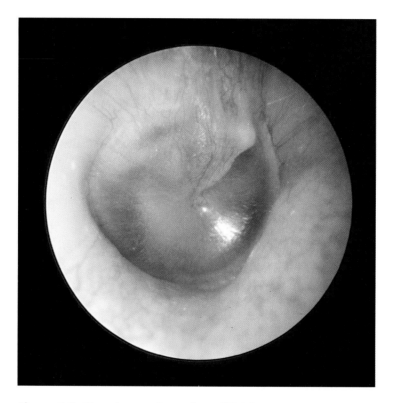

Figure 5.2 Normal tympanic membrane (Right)

In this case the chorda tympani nerve can be clearly seen curving behind the postero-superior quadrant of the tympanic membrane. In addition a leash of vessels can be seen running medially down the superior part of the deep external canal and on to the malleus handle. They are derived from the deep auricular branch of the maxillary artery. They are of variable prominence. This appearance is quite normal.

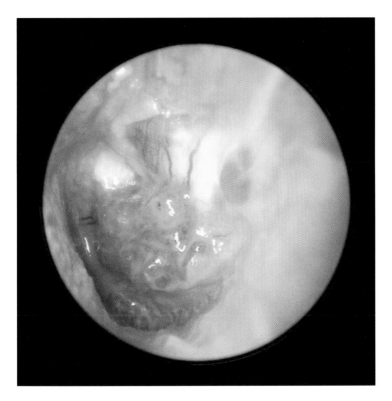

Figure 5.3 Granular myringitis

This condition appears to be due to a chronic infection of the surface layer of the tympanic membrane. A variety of organisms may be responsible and lead to a layer of thickened red granulation tissue over a variable portion of the eardrum. Hearing is impaired and there is frequently discharge from the affected ear. Treatment requires removal of the granulations and topical antibiotic/antifungal and steroid combinations.

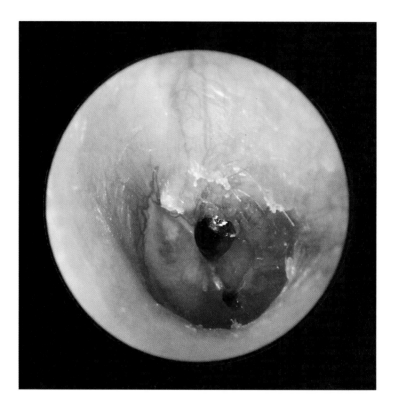

Figure 5.4 Traumatic perforation

Traumatic perforations may be the result of either sudden changes in pressure within the external auditory canal or direct trauma to the tympanic membrane from an inserted implement. In this case it was the result of a blow on the side of the head.

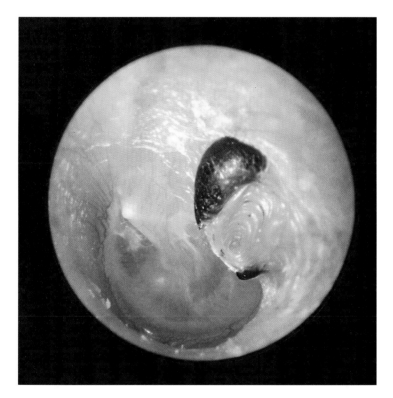

Figure 5.5 Traumatic perforation – healed

As these people usually have normal ears prior to the injury, healing in six to eight weeks is the norm, as has occurred in this case (which is the same as Figure 4.36). If the perforation persists, surgical repair may be required.

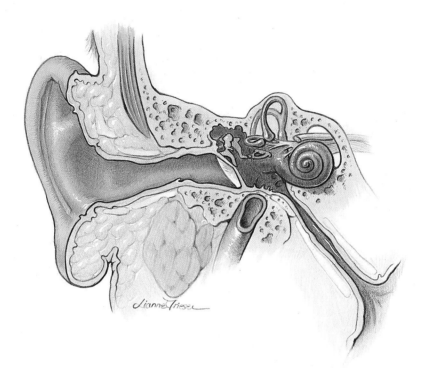

Figure 5.6 Eustachian Tube

The eustachian tube and its function are the key to pathology of the middle ear. The eustachian tube runs from the nasopharynx to the anterior wall of the middle ear cavity. Its lateral third is bony and open, its medial two thirds are cartilaginous and closed. This portion is opened briefly during swallowing by the action of muscles attached to its cartilage skeleton. The function of the eustachian tube is to counteract the continuous absorption of air from the middle ear cleft by aerating and maintaining normal atmospheric pressure within the middle ear. This allows optimal function of the sound transformer mechanism. (*Illustrated by Lianne Friesen*)

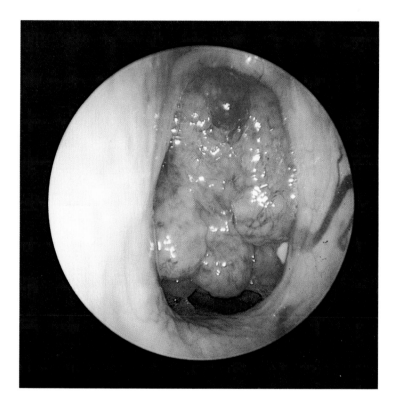

Figure 5.7 Adenoid pad

Eustachian tube function is almost universally impaired in children due to a combination of adenoidal hypertrophy, morphological features and frequent upper respiratory tract infections. These factors account for the high prevalence of middle ear disorders in children. This slide shows a prominent adenoid pad compromising the nasopharyngeal airway.

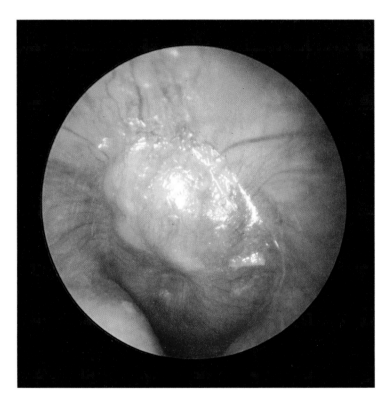

Figure 5.8 Acute otitis media 1

This is almost exclusively a condition of young children and is an acute bacterial
infection of the middle ear cleft. The first changes are usually redness of the drum
and slight swelling, particularly of the upper portion (the pars flaccida).

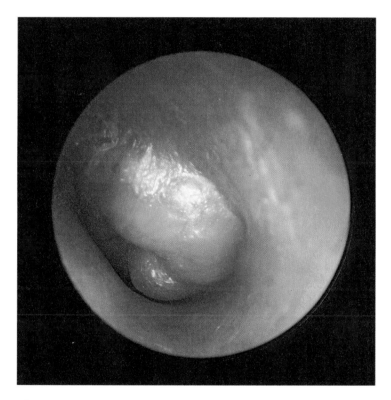

Figure 5.9 Acute otitis media 2

As the condition progresses, the middle ear fills with mucopurulent exudate, causing the drum to bulge laterally.

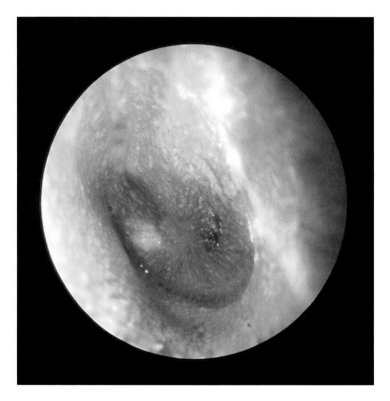

Figure 5.10 Acute otitis media 3

With further progression, a pressure necrosis of the drum may develop, usually posteriorly. This allows a perforation to occur with discharge of the mucopurulent material. Resolution usually follows. This is just about to occur in this drum.

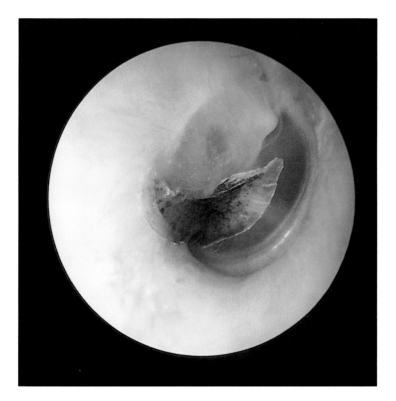

Figure 5.11 Acute otitis media 4

Severe infection in the middle ear can extend into the tympanic membrane and cause a serous transudate through the tympanic membrane. This, mixed with the hyperkeratosis that follows any inflammatory process, leads to the formation of casts on the surface of the drum. This finding therefore serves as an indicator of recent middle ear infection.

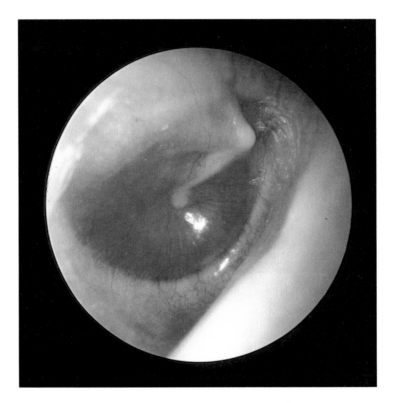

Figure 5.12 Mucoid otitis media (Otitis media with effusion/Glue ear)
This chronic condition results from prolonged eustachian tube dysfunction
leading to a mucoid effusion in the middle ear and is the most common cause of
mild to moderate hearing impairment in children. This slide shows the classical
appearances with a dull appearance to the tympanic membrane and loss of the light
reflex, indicating fluid in the middle ear, and a foreshortening of the malleus handle,
indicating retraction.

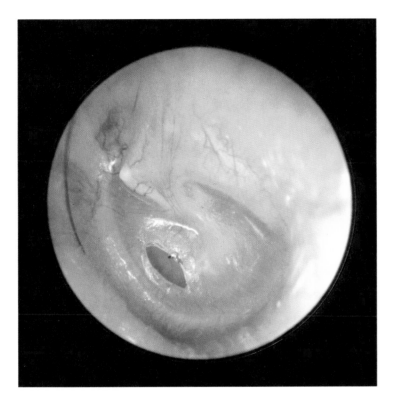

Figure 5.13 Mucoid otitis media 2

Although given enough time (three to four months), most cases will resolve spontaneously and require no treatment, in persistent cases and those with a hearing loss, surgical treatment will be required which involves the insertion of a ventilation tube. The first step in this process is an incision in the eardrum, or myringotomy.

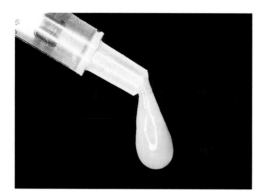

Figure 5.14 Mucoid otitis media 3
The mucoid fluid is then aspirated from the middle ear cleft. This thick opalescent fluid is rich in amino-glycans and inflammatory proteins which give it its "glue-like" consistency.

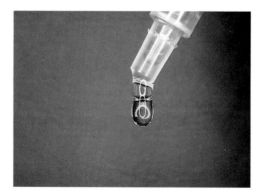

Figure 5.15 Serous otitis media
This is in marked contrast to the thin, yellow, watery fluid obtained by aspiration from the middle ear in serous otitis media.

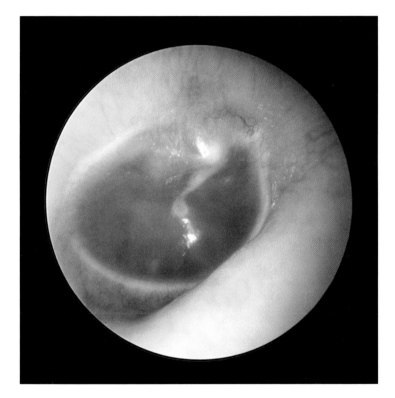

Figure 5.16 Serous otitis media

Serous otitis media occurs as a result of eustachian tube dysfunction or obstruction
in the adult. Its occurrence should always demand a thorough assessment of
the nasopharynx to exclude pathology there. As can be seen here, the thinner fluid
allows much more of the middle ear contents to be seen through the dulled eardrum.

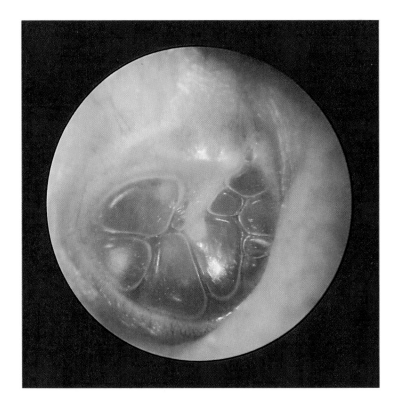

Figure 5.17 Serous otitis media – after auto-inflation

Auto-inflation of the middle ear may be possible in some cases. This is achieved by performing a forced expiration with the mouth and nose closed and literally making one's ears "pop". The air in the middle ear can be seen in the form of bubbles.

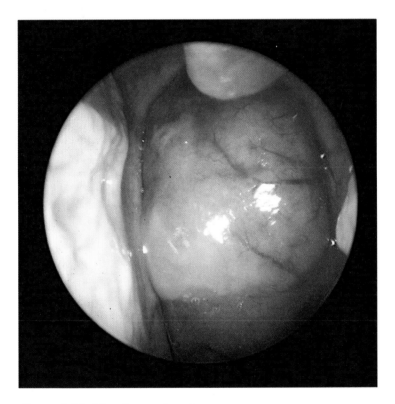

Figure 5.18 Nasopharyngeal carcinoma

Serous otitis media is a common presenting feature of nasopharyngeal carcinoma due to interference with eustachian tube function. In this case the eustachian tube orifice is completely occluded by tumor.

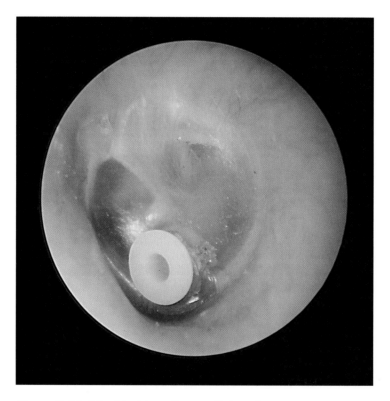

Figure 5.19 Mucoid otitis media – ventilation tube
In this patient a ventilation tube has been inserted into the antero inferior quadrant of the tympanic membrane. This allows continuous aeration of the middle ear and "bypasses" the dysfunctional eustachian tube.

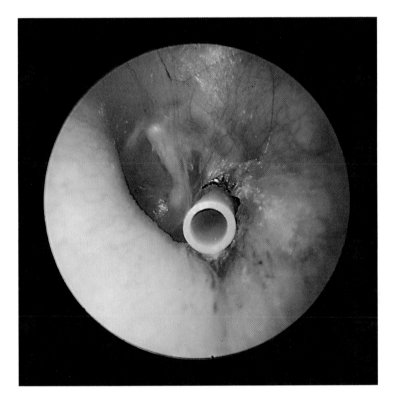

Figure 5.20 Mucoid otitis media – ventilation tube
There are a variety of ventilation tubes available. Most frequently used are the
grommet/bobbin variety (as shown in the previous slide) which have a functional
life of six to twelve months. A T-tube, shown here, tends to have a much longer
functional life, usually measured in years.

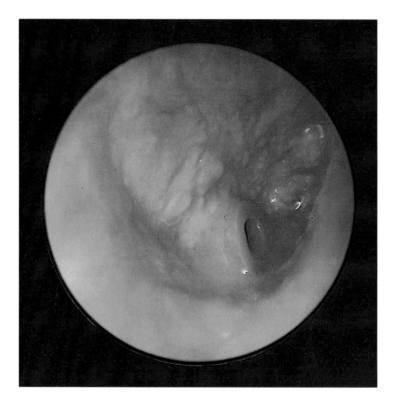

Figure 5.21   Mucoid otitis media – ventilation tube
Infection around a ventilation tube is not uncommon and will usually respond to
topical treatment. If not, it may require removal to resolve the infection.

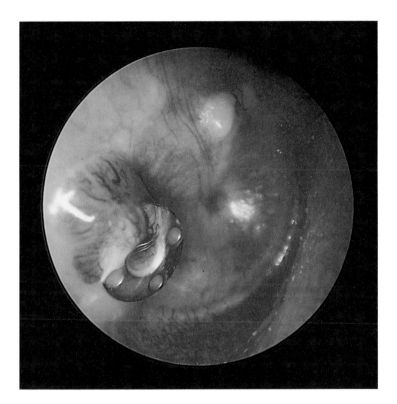

Figure 5.22 Ventilation tube granuloma
Granulation tissue may form around the ventilation tube as a result of local irritation and a keratin foreign body reaction. This may lead to blockage of the tube and discharge from the ear. Topical treatment is again normally sufficient although, in some cases, removal of the tube and its associated granulation tissue may be required.

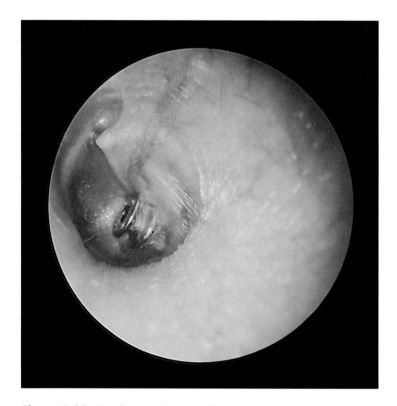

Figure 5.23 Ventilation tube – extruding

In most cases, after a variable period of time, the tube will spontaneously extrude.
Hopefully the affected child will have outgrown the condition although in up to 30
to 40 percent of cases a further set of tubes will be required.

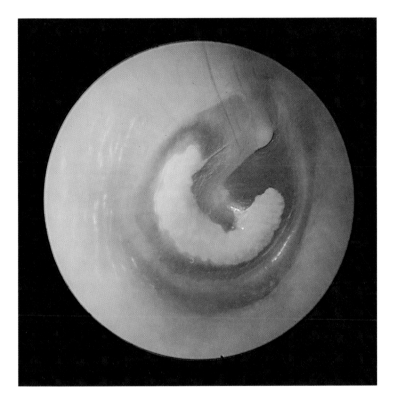

Figure 5.24 Tympanosclerosis

These patches of hyalinization and calcification in the tympanic membrane are commonly associated with the insertion of ventilation tubes (50 to 60 percent). They are thought to be due to a combination of bleeding within the layers of the eardrum at the time of tube insertion and subsequent shear stresses with the tube in place. Note the classic horseshoe shape of the tympanosclerosis.

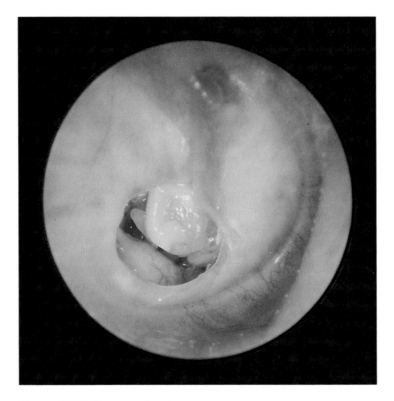

Figure 5.25 Tympanosclerosis

Despite its impressive appearance, tympanosclerosis rarely interferes with hearing. If particularly florid it may extend into the middle ear, resulting in fixation of the ossicles and a conductive hearing loss.

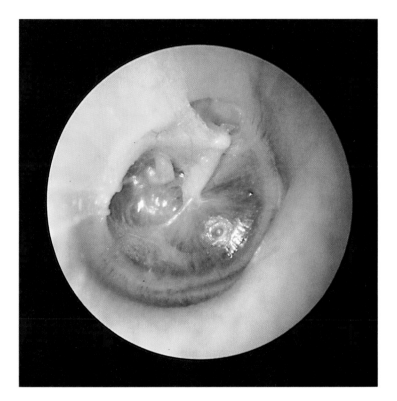

Figure 5.26 Retraction pockets
Although, by the end of childhood, most people will attain normal eustachian tube
function, there is a significant minority for whom this is not so. This group will go
on to develop chronic ear disease as adults. Typically the chronic negative middle
ear pressure will lead to "retraction pockets". In this case there is a retraction of the
postero-superior quadrant of the eardrum which has attached itself to the incudo-
stapedial joint: a myringo-stapediopexy.

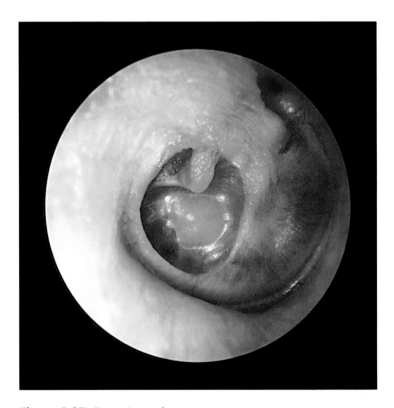

Figure 5.27 Retraction pockets

There is a similar appearance in this case although a larger part of the drum has retracted. Note also the retraction just above the lateral process of the malleus: a so-called attic retraction. In these two cases the process of epithelial migration is able to proceed normally and the retraction pockets are described as "self-cleansing".

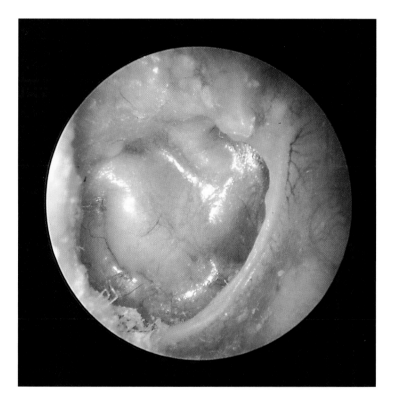

Figure 5.28 Adhesive otitis media

In some unfortunate individuals the whole tympanic membrane may become
retracted and plastered down onto the contents of the middle ear. The ossicles are
frequently eroded and a conductive hearing loss ensues. This is end stage disease
and surgical treatment is usually unrewarding.

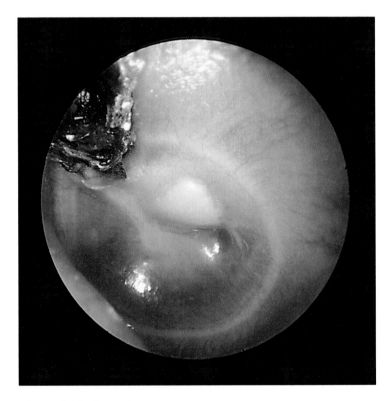

Figure 5.29 Retraction pockets

If the retraction pocket reaches a certain size or configuration, it will no longer be self-cleansing. Keratin debris will build up in the pocket and, by definition, a cholesteatoma has formed. One of the classic pitfalls with cholesteatoma is "attic wax". No examination should be considered complete until the full extent of the tympanic membrane is visualized. Although the attic defect may not look unduly large, cholesteatomas often display extensive infiltration of the middle ear and mastoid system. In this case a large extension into the middle ear cleft can be seen clearly.

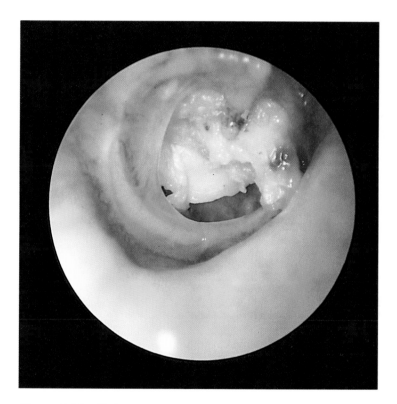

Figure 5.30 Cholesteatoma

This slide shows the classic white cheesy appearance of a cholesteatoma which, in this case is largely filling the middle ear cleft and is seen through a perforated tympanic membrane. The inflammatory process that cholesteatoma incites may lead to bony erosion and the complications of hearing loss, mastoiditis, facial palsy, labyrinthitis, meningitis and brain abscess.

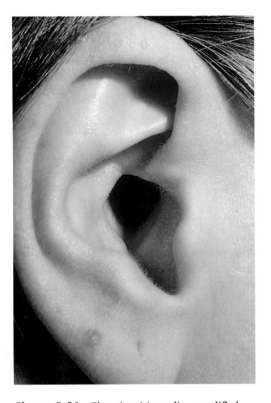

Figure 5.31 Chronic otitis media – modified
radical mastoidectomy – Meatoplasty
In view of the potential complications, surgical treatment of cholesteatoma is indicated in most cases. The
modified radical mastoidectomy shown here has stood
the test of time as a treatment for cholesteatoma. As
part of the operation, the cartilaginous canal is enlarged
to allow better access and aeration of the newly created
mastoid cavity.

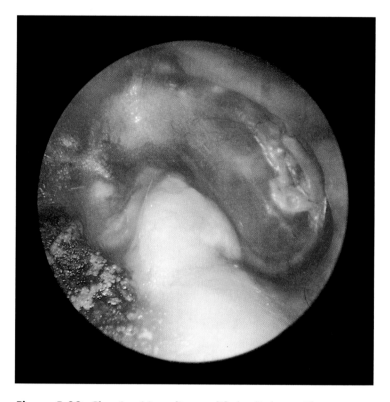

Figure 5.32 Chronic otitis media – modified radical mastoidectomy

This figure shows a typical modified radical mastoidectomy cavity. In this operation
the head of the malleus, the incus, the diseased portion of the tympanic membrane
and mastoid air cells are removed to create a large open cavity.

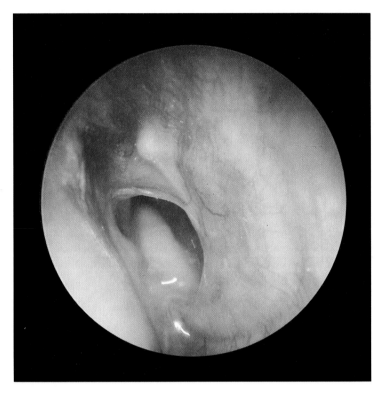

Figure 5.33 Perforation

Chronic or recurrent infection of the middle ear may lead to a perforation of the eardrum which may in turn predispose to further infections. In this case there is a perforation of the eardrum which has granulomatous edges and mucopurulent discharge indicating current infection.

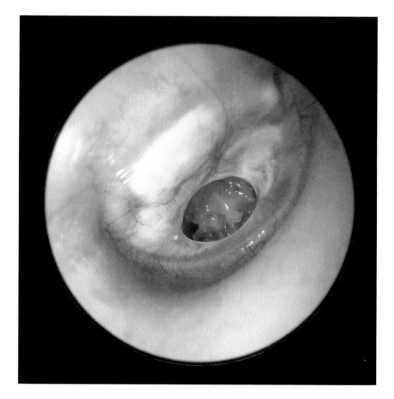

Figure 5.34 Perforation

In this case the perforation is dry and uninfected. It lies in the antero-inferior segment of the drum and as it is completely surrounded by a rim of tympanic membrane, it is therefore described as "central" as opposed to "marginal" where this is not the case. Note the co-existent tympanosclerosis.

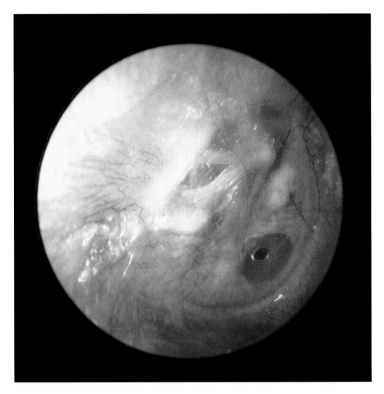

Figure 5.35 Perforation
This would be described as a pinhole perforation.

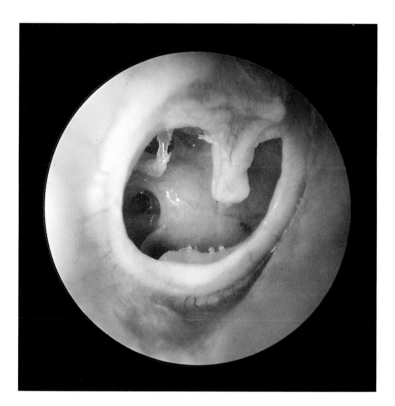

Figure 5.36 Perforation

This would be described as a sub-total perforation for obvious reasons. Note that the incudo-stapedial joint and stapedius tendon are visible through the perforation. There is also some atrophy of the long process of the incus which appears to exist as little more than a fibrous band.

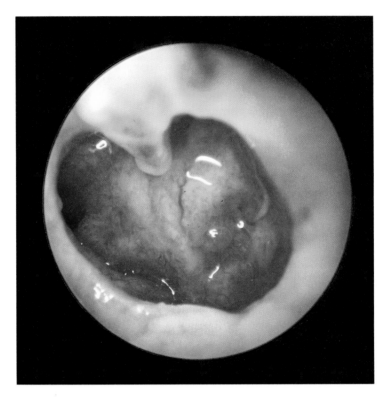

Figure 5.37 Perforation – upper respiratory tract infection

These patients frequently suffer otorrhoea during episodes of upper respiratory tract infection. As can be seen here, this is due to the hyperaemia and excessive mucus production associated with the resulting inflammation of the middle ear mucosa.

Tumors

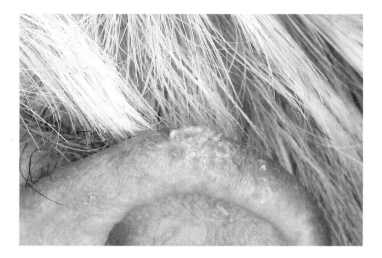

Figure 6.1 Actinic keratosis of pinna

These pre-malignant lesions are common findings on the elderly pinna. They result from chronic sun exposure, and have the propensity to develop into squamous or basal cell carcinoma. Local excision biopsy may be indicated if there is doubt about the diagnosis.

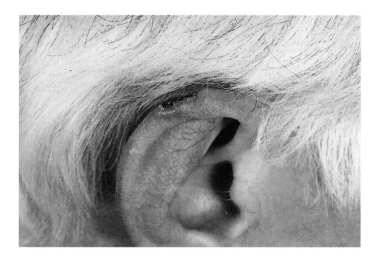

Figure 6.2 Basal cell carcinoma (rodent ulcer) of pinna

Basal cell carcinoma is one of the most common tumors found in the head and neck region. It presents a variety of clinical appearances. Although usually ulcerated, as shown here, it may exist in a "cystic" form. Any suspicious lesions should always be biopsied. Treatment may be by radiotherapy or generous local excision. (*Courtesy of Dr. Peter Adamson*)

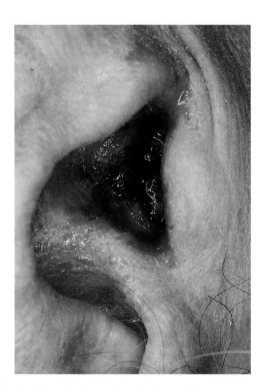

Figure 6.3 Squamous cell carcinoma of pinna
Squamous cell carcinoma is much less common than
basal cell carcinoma. It is nearly always a consequence of
solar damage. Biopsy will again confirm the diagnosis
and treatment is usually by wide local excision.
Squamous cell carcinoma are more aggressive than basal
cell carcinoma.

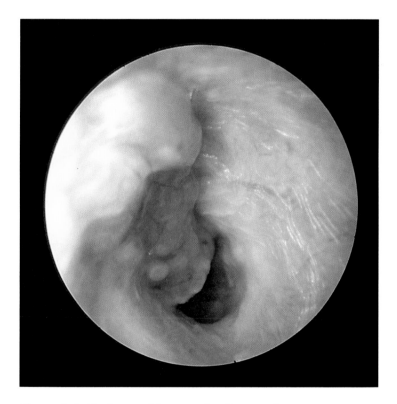

Figure 6.4 Carcinoma of the external auditory canal
While carcinoma of the external canal is extremely uncommon, any granular or
ulcerated lesions in the canal that fail to respond to appropriate treatment or
to heal in a reasonable period of time should always be biopsied. This granular
lesion turned out to be a verrucous carcinoma.

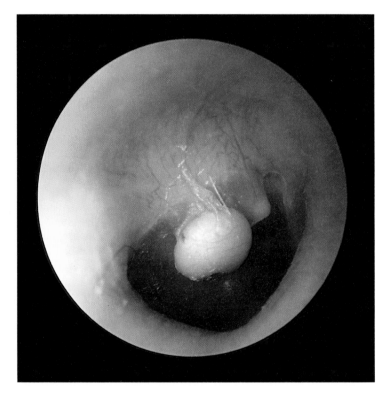

Figure 6.5 Epidermal cyst of the tympanic membrane
During the process of early development, islands of squamous epithelium may become trapped between the outer layers of the tympanic membrane. These benign tumors tend to grow slowly. Their removal is normally straightforward. (*Courtesy of Dr. Jacob Friedberg*)

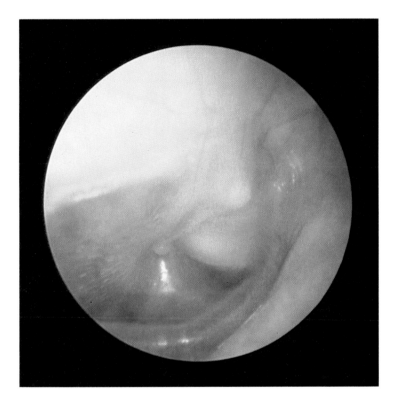

Figure 6.6 Congenital middle ear cholesteatoma

On rare occasions squamous epithelium may become trapped in the middle ear during early development. The result is a slowly growing epidermal cyst, the only indication of which may be as seen here, a white "tumor" seen behind the antero-superior quadrant of the tympanic membrane. (*Courtesy of Dr. Jacob Friedberg*)

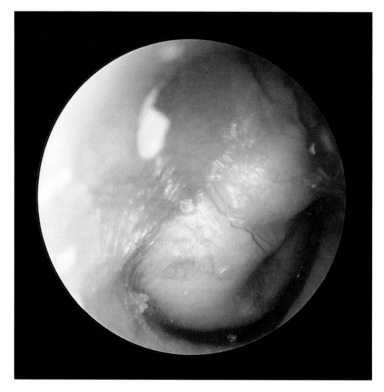

Figure 6.7 Advanced congenital middle ear cholesteatoma
If left untreated, this benign epidermal cyst will slowly enlarge eroding the ossicles
and filling the middle ear cavity. This five-year-old child presented with facial
paralysis as a direct consequence of erosion of the fallopian canal. (*Courtesy of
Dr. Jacob Friedberg*)

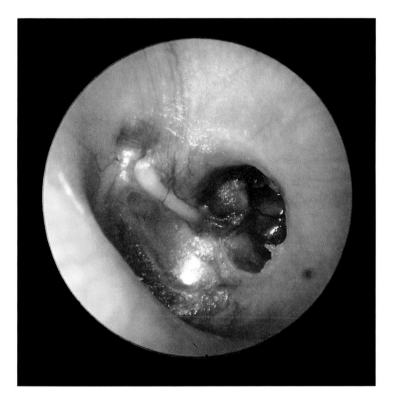

Figure 6.8 Cholesterol granuloma
This uncommon condition is a specific foreign body reaction to cholesterol crystals
found in the middle ear mucosa of patients with chronic ear disease. The color may
vary from yellow to brown.

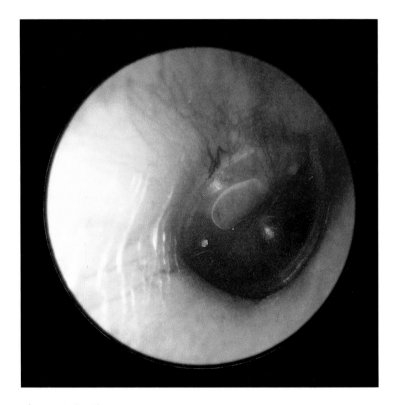

Figure 6.9 Glomus tympanicum

This small red mass seen through the postero-superior quadrant of the tympanic membrane is a tumor of specialized cells arising from the tympanic plexus on the promontory. A tumor of this size may often be removed through a tympanotomy approach.

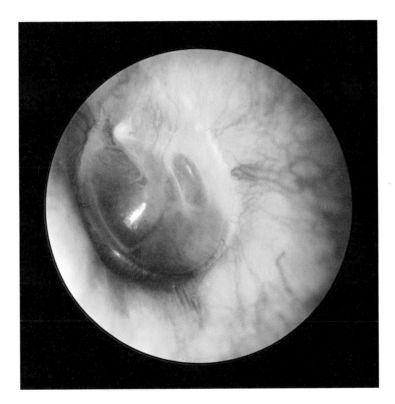

Figure 6.10 Glomus jugulare

This large red mass filling the middle ear and distorting the tympanic membrane is a glomus jugulare tumor. It arises from specialized chemosensory cells found on the jugular bulb. A tumor of this size will require extensive skull base surgery for its removal.

Index